FROM MANAGING TO CONQUERING EPIDIDYMITIS

Expert Guide To Understanding the Causes, Recognizing Symptoms, Prevention and Embracing Effective Treatments for a Vibrant and Healthy Life

DR. DASHIELL DANIEL

Disclaimer

This book, is intended to provide information and guidance on the subject matter and is not a substitute for professional medical advice, diagnosis, or treatment.

The author does not own or endorse any such entities mentioned in the book. Any resemblance to actual persons, living or dead, or actual events is purely coincidental.

Readers are encouraged to consult with qualified healthcare professionals for medical advice, diagnosis, and treatment tailored to their specific circumstances.

The author and the publisher disclaim any liability for any loss or risk, personal or otherwise, arising directly or indirectly from the use of the information presented in this book.

By reading this book, the reader acknowledges and agrees to the terms of this disclaimer.

The book "Epididymitis" is an extensive and invaluable resource that explores the complexities of this illness, offering a complete comprehension of its definition, kinds, causes, and risk factors. Throughout the book, the significance of treating epididymitis is emphasized, along with its significant impact on male reproductive health and the ensuing psychological and emotional fallout. The investigation starts with a thorough analysis of the morphology and physiological functions of the epididymis, explaining its composition, role in the maturation of sperm, and typical operation, encompassing sperm transportation, storage, and hormone control.

The book methodically discusses the symptoms and indicators of epididymitis as the story goes on, providing information on typical symptoms, early warning indicators, and when to seek medical assistance. The entire diagnostic process is covered in detail, including imaging investigations, laboratory testing like blood and urine tests, physical examination methods, and medical histories. A thorough discussion is given to the complex nature of the causes and risk factors of epididymitis, including bacterial infections, non-bacterial causes, and related risk factors like age, demographics, and behavioral variables.

The book delves deeper into therapeutic choices, such as lifestyle changes for all-encompassing care, pain management techniques, and antibiotic treatments aimed at bacterial infections.

The significance of routine testing, safe sexual behaviors, and hygiene considerations are among of the prevention strategies that are addressed. The long-term consequences and possible complications of epididymitis are carefully considered, with a focus on managing chronic patients. There is also discussion of the effect on fertility and the next steps for evaluating and pursuing fertility treatment.

The book addresses the psychological and emotional effects of epididymitis and provides insightful information on coping strategies for chronic pain, mental health issues, and the value of support systems. The study of relationship dynamics emphasizes closeness, communication techniques, and emotional support.

Essentially, this book is an essential academic resource that offers a thorough and detailed analysis of epididymitis, guaranteeing that academics, doctors, and laypeople alike can gain a profound comprehension of the illness and its consequences.

Introduction

The medical disorder known as epididymitis is typified by inflammation of the epididymis, a coiled tube that stores and transports sperm and is situated behind the testicles. Numerous conditions, including as urinary tract infections, bacterial infections, and sexually transmitted infections (STIs), can trigger this inflammation. Given that epididymitis can have serious consequences for the health of male reproduction, understanding it is essential for both management and prevention. The definition, types, causes, and risk factors of epididymitis will all be covered in detail during this topical discussion.

Recognizing Epididymitis

Synopsis and Definition:

The term "epidymitis" describes inflammation of the epididymis, which is an essential part of the male reproductive system and is in charge of storing and maturing sperm. The scrotum may experience pain, swelling, and discomfort as a result of the inflammation. There are two primary categories of epididymitis: acute and chronic. While chronic epididymitis persists over a longer length of time with symptoms that may fluctuate in intensity, acute epididymitis develops rapidly and is frequently caused by bacterial infections.

It is essential to comprehend the nature of epididymitis in order to create focused and efficient treatment plans.

Epididymitis Types

Acute and chronic epididymitis are the two main forms, and they differ in how they begin, last, and have underlying reasons. Most cases of acute epididymitis are caused by bacterial infections, which are frequently the consequence of urinary tract infections or sexually transmitted infections (STIs). Conversely, non-infectious reasons such trauma or autoimmune diseases, recurrent infections, or past episodes of acute epididymitis may be connected to chronic epididymitis. Given that treatment modalities differ, making the distinction between these categories is essential for precise diagnosis and effective intervention.

Reasons And Danger Factors

There are multiple elements involved in the onset of epididymitis. One of the main causes is bacterial infections, which are frequently linked to pathogens such as Neisseria gonorrhoeae, Escherichia coli, and Chlamydia trachomatis. Additionally, inflammation can be brought on by urinary tract infections that reach the epididymis. Unprotected sexual activity, a history of STIs, anatomical anomalies, and urinary catheter use are risk factors for epididymitis. Comprehending these causes and risk factors facilitates preventive actions and educates people about the significance of safe sexual practices and timely medical assistance when pertinent risk factors are present.

The Significance Of Overcoming Epididymitis

Effect on the Health of Male Reproduction:

Since epididymitis has a major effect on the health of male reproduction, its elimination is of utmost importance. Sperm maturation and storage depend heavily on the epididymis, and inflammation can interfere with these processes, resulting in sperm that are not as healthy or functional. Untreated or repeated epididymitis may lead to infertility because impaired sperm may find it difficult to fertilize eggs. In order to reduce the chance of long-term reproductive issues and maintain fertility in those who are impacted, epididymitis must be treated as soon as possible.

Effects On The Mind And Emotions

In addition to its physical consequences, epididymitis can affect a person's mental and emotional state. Anxiety, tension, and a lowered quality of life can be brought on by the pain and suffering this disorder causes. Additionally, worries regarding the health of the reproductive system and fertility might exacerbate mental distress. In addition to medical care, psychological support and counseling are also important components of treating epididymitis because they can negatively impact an individual's mental state and general well-being.

knowledge of the specifics of epididymitis, such as its kinds, definition, causes, and hazards, is essential for both care and prevention. It is imperative to overcome epididymitis in order to protect male reproductive health, avoid problems with conception, and manage the emotional and psychological effects of this illness. All-encompassing approaches that include medical interventions, prophylactic measures, and psychosocial support are critical to the effective management of epididymitis and the enhancement of afflicted individuals' general welfare.

CHAPTER ONE
THE EPIDIDYMIS'S ANATOMY AND OPERATION

As a place for sperm maturation and storage, the epididymis is essential to the male reproductive system. Gaining an understanding of the structure and operation of the epididymis is necessary to appreciate its importance in reproductive health.

The epididymis's structure is carefully crafted to enable its various roles. The epididymis is made up of a tightly wound tubule that is separated into three main sections: the head, body, and tail. Spermatozoa are delivered to the head by the efferent ductules, which are located close to the upper pole of the testis. Sperm go through a number of physiological changes that indicate the change from immature to mature forms when they pass through the epididymis. A favorable milieu for sperm maturation is provided by the pseudostratified columnar epithelium with stereocilia that is a feature of the intricate structure of the epididymis. Furthermore, smooth muscle layers support sperm movement in the epididymal duct.

One essential part of the epididymis's function is its involvement in the maturation of sperm. Sperm undergo many alterations that improve their motility and fertilization capacities as they travel through the epididymal duct. The epididymis provides a milieu that makes it easier to acquire certain proteins, modify the composition of the membrane, and remove extra cytoplasm.

These modifications are necessary to allow sperm to enter the female reproductive system and fertilize eggs. As a result, any alteration to the epididymis's natural structure or function may affect sperm maturation and jeopardize male fertility.

Transport and storage of sperm as well as hormone management are two essential functions of the epididymis in normal functioning.

The influx of spermatozoa from the testis into the epididymis via the efferent ductules marks the start of sperm transport. The epididymal tubule's coiled form creates an environment that is favorable for sperm to proceed gradually. Furthermore, sperm are propelled towards the vas deferens by smooth muscle contractions within the epididymal walls, which ultimately aids in their release during ejaculation. Additionally, the epididymis acts as a reservoir for mature sperm, enabling the preservation of viable spermatozoa until fertilization is required.

Another essential component of the epididymis' regular operation is hormone control.

The hormonal environment, which is mostly regulated by testosterone, is essential for preserving the microenvironment that sperm need to mature. Testosterone has a role in the maturation process by controlling the secretion of several substances within the epididymis, such as proteins and enzymes. The delicate balance necessary for the best possible sperm growth and function might be upset by any imbalance in hormone regulation.

Overcoming epididymitis entails resolving issues with the anatomical and functional features of the epididymis. Normal sperm maturation and transit may be hampered by epididymitis, a condition marked by inflammation of the epididymal duct. Numerous things, such as bacterial infections, trauma, or underlying medical disorders, can cause inflammation. It is crucial to take into account how treating epididymitis would affect the intricate structure of the epididymis. The integrity of the epididymal epithelium may be jeopardized by inflammatory processes, which can also impair smooth muscle activity and produce an unsuitable environment for sperm maturation.

Moreover, changes in hormone regulation may result from the inflammatory reaction linked to epididymitis. Inflammatory mediators have the potential to disrupt the precise hormonal signal balance necessary for the best possible function of the epididym. The inflammatory cascade may have an impact on testosterone, a crucial hormone in this situation, which could cause disruptions in the microenvironment required for sperm development. As a result, treating epididymitis entails not only controlling the inflammatory process but also reestablishing the epididymis's normal anatomical structure and hormonal balance.

Antimicrobial therapy is frequently used to treat epididymitis in order to eradicate the underlying infection. The causative agent determines which antibiotics should be provided, and a detailed knowledge of the anatomy of the epididym is essential to figuring out the best way to distribute the medication and get it into the damaged tissues. In extreme situations, surgery can be required to remove damaged epididymis sections or drain abscesses. Anti-inflammatory drugs may also be used to lessen the inflammatory response and stop more harm to the epididymal tissue.

treating and curing epididymitis requires a thorough grasp of the structure and function of the epididymis. With its complex anatomy and vital function in sperm maturation, the epididymis is a vital part of male reproductive health. Abnormalities in the normal operation of the epididymis, such as epididymitis, can significantly affect the fertility of males. To maintain the best possible reproductive health, treatment strategies must thus not only address the underlying causes but also work to return the epididymis's normal anatomical structures and hormonal balance.

CHAPTER TWO
EPIDIDYMITIS SIGNIFICATIONS AND SYMPTOMS

The signs and symptoms of epididymitis, an inflammatory disease that affects the epididymis, a coiled tube behind the testicles, range in severity. Acknowledging these expressions is essential for prompt action and efficient handling.

Early Warning indicators: Identifying Mild Symptoms: People may exhibit mild symptoms in the early stages of epididymitis. If these indicators are promptly recognized, early care can be beneficial. One of the milder symptoms could be a slight scrotal soreness or discomfort that is frequently written off as irrelevant or transient.

But, attention is essential since, if ignored, these early symptoms could worsen.

When to Seek Medical assistance: The key to successfully treating epididymitis is knowing when to seek medical assistance. Patients should be made aware of the significance of seeking medical attention from a professional if they are in pain for an extended period of time, as failure to do so may result in consequences. Prompt medical care guarantees not only immediate relief but also stops the illness from worsening.

Common Symptoms: Pain and Discomfort: Pain and discomfort are two of the most common signs of epididymitis. Usually starting in the afflicted testicle, the pain can range in intensity from a subtle aching to a strong stabbing feeling. Comprehensive pain management techniques are required because this discomfort may get worse when exercising or peeing.

edema and Inflammation: Notable scrotal edema and redness are a result of the inflammatory nature of epididymitis. Determining the causes underlying this swelling is essential to creating tailored treatment strategies.

Increased blood flow and fluid buildup can cause swelling, which highlights the necessity of anti-inflammatory treatments to lessen these symptoms.

Other accompanying Symptoms: In addition to localized symptoms, a variety of accompanying systemic symptoms can also be present with epididymitis. For example, fever may be present along with the illness, indicating a more extensive immunological response.

Further complicating the clinical picture are urine symptoms that patients may suffer, such as dysuria or frequency.

These accompanying symptoms call for a thorough evaluation to determine the severity of the illness and inform the most effective course of treatment.

both individuals and healthcare providers need to have a sophisticated grasp of the indications and manifestations of epididymitis. The course of the disease can be greatly impacted by early detection of modest symptoms and aggressive seeking of medical assistance.

It is important to carefully assess common symptoms including pain, edema, and related systemic manifestations in order to customize therapies that address the complex character of epididymitis.

CHAPTER THREE
EPIDIDYMITIS DIAGNOSIS

The inflammation of the epididymis, a coiled tube that stores and transports sperm at the back of the testicles, is the hallmark of the clinical illness epididymitis. For problems to be effectively managed and prevented, an accurate diagnosis is essential. A thorough approach is used in the diagnostic procedure, which includes laboratory testing, imaging investigations, physical examinations, and assessments of medical histories.

Medical Background Information And Physical Assessment

A complete medical history and physical examination are necessary in order to make the initial diagnosis of epididymitis. Healthcare providers obtain vital information about the patient's symptoms, when they first appeared, and any possible risk factors, like recent sexual activity or urinary tract infections, during the patient interview (4.1.1). This thorough history helps determine probable causes and customize further diagnostic procedures.

Techniques for physical examination (4.1.2) are essential to the diagnosis procedure. Examining the genitalia carefully, clinicians palpate the scrotum to feel for edema and soreness. Inflammation is indicated by erythema, warmth, and swelling in the epididymis area.

The examination may also involve evaluating the patient's inguinal and abdominal regions in order to rule out additional potential sources of pain and discomfort.

Lab Examinations

To confirm the diagnosis of epididymitis and determine the underlying cause, laboratory testing are necessary. A crucial diagnostic technique is urinalysis (4.2.1), which aids in identifying bacteria, white blood cells, and other anomalies in the urine. A positive urine culture for bacteria can direct antibiotic therapy and provide important information about the causing organism.

To measure inflammatory indicators including C-reactive protein (CRP) and white blood cell count, blood tests (4.2.2) may be performed. Increased levels of these markers can show how severe the inflammatory response is and help confirm the diagnosis of epididymitis.

Imaging Research

To see the epididymis and associated structures, imaging investigations (4.2.3) are frequently utilized. This helps with diagnosis confirmation and evaluation of potential problems. The preferred imaging modality is ultrasound since it provides a thorough and non-invasive evaluation of the scrotum. It may show enlargement of the epididymis, elevated blood flow, abscesses, or other problems.

the procedure of diagnosing epididymitis is complex and includes a thorough physical examination and medical history, in addition to laboratory tests and imaging examinations. Healthcare providers can make an accurate diagnosis, identify the underlying reason, and start timely, focused treatment plans because to the integration of many diagnostic modalities.

CHAPTER FOUR
FACTORS OF RISK AND CAUSES

An inflammation of the epididymis, a coiled tube behind the testicles that stores and transports sperm, is the hallmark of the medical illness epididymitis. Gaining control over epididymitis necessitates a thorough comprehension of its causes and risk factors, with an emphasis on risk factors that are related to both bacterial and non-bacterial sources.

Significant subgroups of urinary tract infections (UTIs) and sexually transmitted infections (STIs) are among the major causes of epididymitis that are attributed to bacterial infections.

Sexually transmitted infections are frequently responsible for the development of epididymitis, including gonorrhea and chlamydia.

Unprotected sexual contact is usually the source of these infections, as it allows the germs to pass through the reproductive system and infect the epididymis. Similarly, when germs from the urinary system climb through the vas deferens to reach the epididymis, urinary tract infections can result in epididymitis.

In order to develop appropriate treatment techniques, which frequently involve antibiotics targeted at the particular pathogenic organisms, it is imperative to understand the microbiological etiology.

Non-bacterial variables are also important in the development of epididymitis in addition to bacterial ones. Both acute and chronic trauma and injuries can cause the epididymis to become inflamed. Accidents, sports-related injuries, or direct trauma to the genital area can all cause this.

Inflammation can also be a symptom of autoimmune diseases, in which the immune system of the body mistakenly targets and attacks the tissues of the penis. Clinicians must comprehend non-bacterial causes in order to develop a comprehensive treatment plan because the therapies used may not be the same as those used for bacterially produced epididymitis.

There are a number of risk factors that increase the chance of acquiring epididymitis.

Demographics and age are important factors, as some age groups are more prone to this illness than others. Teenagers and young adults are more vulnerable, particularly when they participate in high-risk activities like unprotected sexual engagement. Multiple sexual partners and inconsistent condom use are two behavioral risk factors that lead to the higher incidence of epididymitis.

Because bacterial causes and behavioral patterns may overlap, it's critical to address both behavioral and microbiological factors in preventive efforts.

treating epididymitis requires a comprehensive knowledge of its risk factors and etiology.

A multifaceted approach to diagnosis, treatment, and prevention is required due to the interaction between bacterial and non-bacterial sources, as well as demographic and behavioral risk factors. In order to effectively manage and combat epididymitis, healthcare providers must have a thorough awareness of these ideas.

CHAPTER FIVE
AVAILABLE TREATMENTS

The ailment known as epididymitis, which is defined by inflammation of the epididymis, frequently requires all-encompassing treatment methods in order to address the underlying causes of the condition and its symptoms. Antibiotic therapy is a fundamental intervention strategy that is used to treat epididymitis.

As a common etiological cause of epididymal inflammation, bacterial infections are the focus of this therapy approach. Antibiotic use attempts to eradicate the bacteria causing the illness and stop it from getting worse or coming back. Antibiotic susceptibility, the particular bacterial strain causing the infection, and the patient's medical history all play a role in the choosing of antibiotics.

Targeting bacterial infections in the context of antibiotic therapy requires a sophisticated understanding in order to effectively intervene. Bacteria that travel via the urinary tract and reach the epididymis frequently cause ascending infections, which lead to epididymitis. As a result, doctors usually prescribe antibiotics that are effective against common urogenital pathogens like Chlamydia trachomatis and Escherichia coli. To maximize treatment results, the antibiotic regimen must be customized to the particular bacterial strain involved. This tailored strategy reduces the possibility of antibiotic resistance and increases the possibility of completely eliminating the infection.

Because of their effectiveness against urogenital bacteria, a number of antibiotics are commonly used in the treatment of epididymitis. Fluoroquinolones, such levofloxacin and ciprofloxacin, are frequently given because of their efficient tissue penetration and broad-spectrum activity. Furthermore, macrolides such as azithromycin are used, especially when Chlamydia trachomatis is suspected. The patient's medical history, including any allergies and possible side effects, is taken into account while selecting antibiotics. Effective antibiotic treatment reduces the likelihood of consequences like the development of an abscess or long-term epididymal damage in addition to treating the acute infection.

Managing Pain In Epididymitis

Since pain is a common and upsetting symptom of epididymitis, it is important to control pain effectively in order to improve patient comfort and quality of life while undergoing therapy.

For those who are suffering from mild to moderate epididymitis pain, over-the-counter drugs are an accessible choice. Nonsteroidal anti-inflammatory medications (NSAIDs), such naproxen and ibuprofen, are often used because of their ability to simultaneously reduce inflammation and discomfort. By preventing the formation of prostaglandins, these drugs reduce inflammation and ease discomfort.

Prescription choices are necessary when over-the-counter drugs are unable to provide appropriate pain relief. Under under medical supervision, opioids like tramadol or oxycodone may be recommended for the treatment of severe pain related to epididymitis. However, because of the risk of reliance and negative effects, using opioids requires careful supervision. Prescriptions for painkillers are only issued after a comprehensive evaluation of the patient's medical history, level of pain, and the overall risk-benefit profile of the selected analgesic.

Non-pharmacological methods are just as important for managing pain in patients with epididymitis as pharmacological ones.

Heat therapy can provide localized relief by increasing blood circulation and lowering muscle tension in the affected area. Examples of this include warm compresses and sitz baths.

Modifications to one's physical activities, such as avoiding activities that make pain worse, can also help manage pain.

Pain management for epididymitis can be achieved by a comprehensive and patient-centered strategy utilizing a combination of pharmacological and non-pharmacological therapies.

Changes In Lifestyle In Epididymitis

A vital part of controlling epididymitis is incorporating lifestyle improvements in addition to medication therapies. In the context of epididymal inflammation, it is critical to understand the significance of rest and relaxation. Getting enough sleep enables the body to focus its efforts on recuperation and mending, which expedites the treatment of symptoms. Restrictions on physical activity may be advised in the acute phase of epididymitis in order to avoid aggravating the condition and speed up the healing process.

A range of lifestyle modifications are included in supportive interventions with the goal of enhancing general well-being and lowering the risk of repeated episodes. In cases when epididymitis is secondary to sexually transmitted infections, maintaining good genital hygiene is essential to preventing its worsening. In order to reduce their risk of contracting infections again, patients are frequently counseled on the significance of safe sexual behavior. Additionally, maintaining a balanced diet and drinking plenty of water help to support the immune system, which strengthens the body's defenses against illnesses.

It's important to include the psychosocial support component of lifestyle alterations as well.

The pain and discomfort that come with epididymitis can have a serious effect on a person's mental health. Improving psychological distress and offering coping skills to patients improves the way the illness is managed overall.

A comprehensive framework for treating epididymitis holistically is created by collaborating between patients and healthcare providers to achieve lifestyle changes, with an emphasis on both the physical and psychological components of therapy.

treating epididymitis requires a multimodal strategy that includes pain relief, antibiotic medication, and lifestyle changes. Effective management of epididymitis requires a full grasp of bacterial targeting in antibiotic therapy, prudent use of pain relievers, and significant lifestyle modifications. These measures enable a patient-centered and holistic approach. Combining these different elements improves the general health of those with this inflammatory disease while also treating the acute symptoms and reducing the chance of recurrence.

CHAPTER SIX
STRATEGIES FOR PREVENTION
Safe Sexual Behavior

The prevention of epididymitis, a disorder characterized by inflammation of the epididymis, a tubular tissue that is essential to the male reproductive system, is greatly aided by safe sexual practices. Avoiding risky activities that could result in sexually transmitted infections (STIs) is a vital component of safe sexual practices. Having several partners during unprotected sexual encounters raises the risk of STIs, which can then result in epididymitis.

To lower the risk of contracting epididymitis, people should prioritize using barrier techniques like condoms to prevent the spread of STIs.

In the context of prevention, the significance of routine STI testing cannot be emphasized, in addition to the adoption of preventative measures. Regular screening helps to identify infections early and treat them quickly, which stops the development of diseases like epididymitis.

The importance of routine STI testing should be emphasized by healthcare professionals, especially for people who participate in high-risk sexual practices. This proactive approach enhances both public and individual health and makes a substantial contribution to the entire prevention strategy.

Practices Of Hygiene
Tips For Personal Hygiene

One crucial element of the multimodal strategy to prevent epididymitis is good personal cleanliness. There are a number of personal hygiene practices that people can follow to reduce their risk of epididymal irritation and infection. It is essential to practice regular and comprehensive genital hygiene, which includes cleaning the vaginal area with a mild soap and water.

Maintaining genital hygiene delays the development of epididymitis by lowering the risk of bacterial growth and infection.

Additionally, people need to be very mindful of their urinal hygiene. To avoid bacteria entering the urethra and climbing up to the epididymis, it is important to keep the urethra clean during urination. It's also important to drink enough water because it encourages frequent urination and aids in clearing the urinary system of any possible infections. In order to enable people to take proactive steps to protect their reproductive health, education on basic personal hygiene habits is essential.

Clothes And Environmental Factors

In addition to maintaining good personal hygiene, clothes and environmental factors play a major role in preventing epididymitis. Wearing loose-fitting underwear that is preferably made of breathable materials helps to keep the genital area less moist and helps to maintain the ideal temperature.

This is especially crucial because warm, humid conditions can encourage the growth of bacteria and raise the risk of epididymitis.

Therefore, choosing clothes with appropriate ventilation and moisture management might be seen as a preventive step.

Environmental considerations should also include things like exposure to allergies or irritants.

People should stay away from anything that could irritate their genital area, such as certain materials or chemicals. In addition, keeping one's living space tidy and sanitary helps reduce exposure to possible infections, which is a supplement to good personal hygiene habits. To effectively avoid epididymitis, a comprehensive strategy that takes into account environmental and personal factors is essential.

a thorough approach that takes into account proper cleanliness and safe sexual behavior is necessary to prevent epididymitis.

A strong preventive framework is formed by highlighting the significance of protective measures during sexual activity, routine STI testing, personal hygiene advice, and environmental factors. Campaigns to raise awareness and educate people are essential for spreading this knowledge, enabling them to take preventative action and lower the prevalence of epididymitis in their communities.

CHAPTER SEVEN
INTRICACIES AND PROLONGED CONSEQUENCES

The inflammation of the epididymis known as epididymitis can have a major negative influence on an affected person's health and well-being due to a number of potential consequences and long-term implications. The emergence of chronic epididymitis, a disorder marked by ongoing inflammation that lasts longer than six weeks, is one of the main worries. Recurrent infections or acute epididymitis that is not effectively treated are common causes of chronic instances. Unresolved predisposing diseases, underlying anatomical defects, and bacterial resistance to antibiotics can all have an impact on the transition to chronicity.

Prolonged Epididymitis

The complicated clinical picture of chronic epididymitis is characterized by recurring scrotal pain and discomfort.

In contrast to acute epididymitis, which usually presents with more prominent symptoms, chronic instances can present with dull or sporadic discomfort, which can complicate diagnosis. People with chronic epididymitis may have physical and psychological distress due to its extended nature, which can have a substantial negative impact on their quality of life.

To customize effective therapeutic techniques, it is imperative to distinguish between various scrotal diseases and chronic epididymitis.

Comprehending Chronic Cases

Understanding the underlying etiology and contributing factors is essential to get a complete understanding of chronic epididymitis. The chronic nature of the illness can also be attributed to non-infectious processes such autoimmune reactions, vasculitis, or nerve entrapment, although bacterial infections are still a prominent cause. Finding the underlying causes is largely dependent on imaging scans, blood work, and thorough patient history reviews. To create complete treatment strategies, urologists, infectious disease specialists, and pain management professionals frequently need to work together in a multidisciplinary manner.

Techniques Of Management

A customized approach that takes into account both the infectious and non-infectious elements of the illness is necessary for the management of chronic epididymitis. In cases when the bacteria are persistently involved, antibiotics may still be useful, but in order to combat antibiotic resistance, the selection of drugs should be based on culture and sensitivity data. Physical therapy, scrotal support, and localized heating treatments are examples of non-pharmacological approaches that can improve patient comfort and reduce discomfort.

Analgesics and anti-inflammatory drugs are two examples of chronic pain management techniques that should be used carefully to balance pain relief with any adverse effects.

Effect On The Rate Of Fertility

Impacts on male fertility are among the major issues raised by epididymitis, especially in chronic cases. A disturbance in the epididymis's function can result in lower-quality sperm since it is essential to the maturation and storage of sperm. Prolonged inflammation can cause scar tissue to develop, which prevents sperm from passing through during ejaculation.

Furthermore, the inflammatory environment in the epididymis might negatively impact the motility and viability of sperm. These elements work together to reduce a person's chance for conception, which emphasizes how critical it is to treat epididymitis as soon as possible.

Evaluating Fertility Problems

When assessing fertility problems in people with a history of epididymitis, a thorough examination of both male and female partners is necessary. Semen analysis, which focuses on factors including sperm count, motility, and morphology, is still the mainstay for evaluating male fertility. Specialized testing, such as sperm DNA fragmentation assays and sperm function tests, may offer greater insights into the effect of epididymitis on sperm quality than simple semen analysis. To evaluate these findings and develop focused fertility therapies, urologists and reproductive experts must work together.

Looking For Treatment For Fertility

Getting fertility treatment becomes an option for couples with chronic epididymitis-related infertility issues. Certain obstacles caused by low-quality sperm can be overcome by assisted reproductive technologies (ART), such as intracytoplasmic sperm injection (ICSI) and in vitro fertilization (IVF). But the effectiveness of fertility therapies for infertility caused by epididymitis depends on a number of variables, such as the degree of sperm abnormalities and the general reproductive health of the female spouse. A key element of the holistic approach to care is providing couples navigating reproductive treatments with counseling and support.

untreated or insufficiently treated epididymitis can result in long-term issues that have a significant impact on reproductive and physical health.

A thorough understanding of the pathogenesis of chronic epididymitis, careful management techniques, and a proactive approach to evaluating and treating reproductive difficulties are all necessary. In order to minimize the long-term repercussions of epididymitis and guarantee the best possible outcomes for afflicted individuals and couples hoping to start a family, prompt and coordinated actions by medical specialists are crucial.

CHAPTER EIGHT
THE IMPACT OF EMOTION AND PSYCHOLOGY

Inflammation of the epididymis is the hallmark of epididymitis, an illness that can have a significant emotional and psychological impact on a person. One of the most important aspects of the patient's experience becomes managing the chronic pain linked to this ailment. As people deal with the difficulties of chronic pain, mental health issues become increasingly important, necessitating a comprehensive strategy to treat both the physical and emotional effects of the condition.

The psychological effect may show up as irritation, despair, or anxiety, which can have an influence on the affected person's general wellbeing.

Handling Prolonged Pain

Managing persistent discomfort linked to epididymitis necessitates a comprehensive strategy.

Patients frequently struggle with bodily discomfort that goes beyond what is strictly medical. Coping mechanisms including mindfulness, cognitive-behavioral therapy, and pain management approaches become essential parts of the process. The psychological effects of chronic pain necessitate a thorough comprehension of the mind-body relationship, highlighting the requirement for specialized interventions that take into account the condition's mental and physical aspects.

Considering Mental Health

The issues related to mental health that arise with epididymitis are diverse. The chronic nature of the illness might aggravate anxiety and depression, which could result in a vicious cycle of increasing psychological anguish and pain perception.

It becomes essential to incorporate mental health assistance into the overall treatment strategy, with medical personnel attending to both physical and emotional issues.

In order to properly treat the emotional impact of epididymitis, patients benefit from a coordinated strategy that includes psychoeducation, counseling, and, when necessary, pharmaceutical interventions.

Assistance Networks

Creating and sustaining support systems is essential to overcoming epididymitis.

Through support groups or online forums, patients can connect with people who have experienced similar things and find peace in that. In the support system, family and friends are essential because they offer both practical and emotional support during trying times.

Throughout the recovery process, healthcare providers should aggressively urge patients to interact with these networks, realizing their importance in reducing feelings of loneliness and promoting a sense of community.

Relationship Dynamics

Relationship dynamics can be greatly impacted by epididymitis, making a nuanced approach to communication and emotional support necessary. While they work to comprehend and support the person with the condition, partners may find themselves in unfamiliar ground. In order to ensure that both parties feel heard and validated in their experiences, it becomes imperative that partners use clear and open communication tactics.

Techniques Of Communication

When it comes to addressing the effects of epididymitis on relationships, effective communication techniques are essential.

The disease presents both physical and emotional issues that partners need to discuss honestly and openly. Talking about therapy plans, addressing issues, and expressing emotional needs are all included in this. In addition, spouses should be actively involved in the treatment process by healthcare providers.

This collaborative approach fosters understanding and mutual support.

Closeness And Emotional Assistance

The condition epididymitis may make intimacy difficult in partnerships. The personal components of the partnership may be impacted by the physical and emotional strain. Couples must work through these issues jointly, giving emotional support first priority and figuring out new, intimate connection opportunities. Healthcare providers should offer advice on how to be intimate while honoring the condition's physical restrictions.

Maintaining a healthy intimate relationship requires finding activities that you both enjoy that don't make you feel more uncomfortable physically and placing a strong emphasis on emotional intimacy.

SUMMARY

treating epididymitis holistically and thoroughly means taking care of not just the physical symptoms but also the psychological and emotional effects on people and their relationships. Building strong support systems and having a sophisticated awareness of mental health issues are essential to managing chronic pain. Relationship dynamics—in particular, intimacy and communication techniques—are crucial to the general wellbeing of those with epididymitis. Healthcare providers can empower patients and their spouses to negotiate the challenges together by identifying and addressing the many facets of this condition. This fosters resilience and promotes holistic healing.

www.ingramcontent.com/pod-product-compliance
Lightning Source LLC
Chambersburg PA
CBHW071129260726
48661CB00006B/2734